To
John
with my
compliments
Julian P. Donahue

SCABIES

BY

KENNETH MELLANBY
C.B.E., Sc.D., F.I.Biol.

Sometime Sorby Research Fellow of the Royal Society of London and Reader in Medical Entomology in the London School of Hygiene and Tropical Medicine

———

Director, Monks Wood Experimental Station, Huntingdon

E. W. CLASSEY LTD.
1972

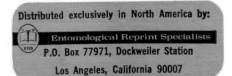

E. W. CLASSEY LTD.
353 Hanworth Road
Hampton
Middlesex TW12 3EN

ISBN 0 900848 61 8

Second Edition
1972

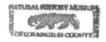
PRINTED IN GREAT BRITAIN BY
BIDDLES LTD., MARTYR ROAD, GUILDFORD

PREFACE

THIS book was first issued in 1943 as one of a series of 'Oxford War Manuals' which dealt with medical problems of importance at that time. Scabies was then a very common complaint, diagnosis was not always accurate, and many patients spent weeks or even months in hospital often suffering from over-treatment with irritant medicants. The book contained the results of research I had recently done, in which I had the willing co-operation of a group of volunteers, who allowed themselves to be exposed to the conditions which we thought, at the outset, would cause them to become infected with the disease. I also had the benefit of very fruitful co-operation with military and civil authorities, with the school medical service, and with many of the leading dermatologists of that period.

After the 1939–45 war, scabies became very rare, and some medical students completed their courses without seeing a single case. However, during the last ten years there has been a considerable increase in the incidence of the disease, as shewn, for instance in the 1970 report on the subject prepared by the Standing Medical Advisory Committee for the Central Health Services Council. Many dermatologists and physicians have told me that they still find their copies of the 1943 edition useful, and that they believe that others would welcome a reprint. I am therefore grateful to Mr. E. W. Classey for making this possible.

In these days of rapid scientific progress, it may seem surprising to re-issue a book of this kind virtually unchanged after 30 years. However, this subject (probably because of the low incidence of scabies) has been almost entirely neglected, and I can find little important new material. The only new clinical complication is one to which my attention has been drawn by Dr. Roderick Howell, Consulting Dermatologist in Swansea. Whereas in 'the old days' we often saw cases in which all the parasites had been killed, but where repeated treatments with potent and irritant medicants (given because the continued itching gave the wrong impression that living

iii

mites were still present) was responsible for an intractable dermatitis, today the situation is different. Secondarily infected scabies cases may be treated with corticosteroids and local applications of antibiotics, so improving the inflammatory and infective aspects of the rash, without the underlying parasites being killed. Such cases are very difficult to diagnose except by actually finding the mites.

When this book was first issued, drugs were scarce and adequate medicants were not always commercially available. This explains the inclusion of details for preparing benzyl benzoate emulsions. These will still be found to be effective, but most physicians will probably use one of the several proprietary brands. It is interesting to note that the price quoted in my 1943 edition for such preparations is slightly *higher* than that charged today. The Pharmaceutical Industry must therefore be congratulated in its contribution in the fight against inflation as well as that against irritation.

Many people have asked me why I think scabies has again become quite a common complaint. Actually I suggested, in 1945, that I expected some sort of an epidemic in another 20–25 years. I based this on the observation that it was much more difficult to reinfect a former patient than to establish an infestation in a new one. In such new cases no irritation or other clinical symptoms appeared for several weeks, during which time a substantial population of mites could develop, and the higher this population the greater the chance of transmission. When reinfections did occur, mite populations were small. This, and the unfamiliarity of both doctors and patients with the disease, could explain its cyclical patterns. As is shewn in this book, dirtiness is not a prime cause, and while increased sexual promiscuity may contribute to the spread in young adults, I think the difference in skin reaction and parasitology is the main cause of the present outbreak.

KENNETH MELLANBY

Monks Wood Experimental Station
September, 1972.

CONTENTS

ILLUSTRATIONS

CHAPTER I

THE ANATOMY AND LIFE HISTORY OF THE ITCH MITE

THE condition known as Scabies or 'the itch' is caused by an invasion of the cuticle of man by the mite *Sarcoptes scabiei* de G. var *hominis*. It was generally held until about a hundred years ago that the disease was caused by some internal metabolic upset, and that although the presence of *Sarcoptes* could sometimes be demonstrated by the expert, the mite was not the primary cause of the disease but either a harmless commensal or a secondary invader. This is not entirely unreasonable, when one considers how widespread are the lesions in many cases and how small is the number of parasites. Another view which has been suggested is that *Sarcoptes*, like so many bacteria, is a normal inhabitant of undiseased skin. Neither of these views will survive investigation. If this parasite invades the cuticle of man, and succeeds in establishing itself, symptoms of scabies will eventually make their appearance, though there may be what is virtually an incubation period during which the acarus will exist in the cuticle without causing any discomfort to the host. During this period it is possible to demonstrate the presence of *Sarcoptes* in the absence of symptoms of scabies, so that the idea that the mite is a mere commensal has some apparent foundation. This symptomless incubation period is, however, of strictly limited duration, though it may extend for several weeks, and once *Sarcoptes* is established the onset of clinical scabies is inevitable. Without the mite, the disease cannot develop, and extermination of the parasite will put an end to the symptoms, though the delay in their total disappearance has given colour to the erroneous belief that scabies can develop without *Sarcoptes*.

Sarcoptes scabiei attacks many different mammals, including dogs, cattle, pigs, sheep, goats, camels, rabbits and horses. No definite morphological distinctions have been described for the *Sarcoptes* found on these different animals, but they nevertheless appear to show physiological distinctions so that the mite from the horse, for instance, though able to attack man, does not usually produce a permanent infestation. It is considered that each mammal has its own peculiar biological race, differing from the *Sarcoptes* from another species in physiology but not in morphology. The life-history of the different races is identical but the reactions of the hosts are not uniform, so that 'sarcoptic mange' in domestic animals is quite unlike human scabies.

Various stages in the life-history of *Sarcoptes* are depicted in Figs. 1 and 2. These drawings were made from specimens taken from human patients suffering from scabies. The adult female (Fig. 1) is the form most commonly seen and most easily isolated from a patient. It is approximately 400 microns (about $\frac{1}{60}$ of an inch) in length. The animal is oval, flat below and convex above. The mounted specimens usually seen and figured in text-books (as Figs. 1*a* and *b*) do not suggest the rounded appearance of the living animal (Fig. 1*c*) and the very striking series of bristles which in certain views are almost reminiscent of those of a hedgehog. There is no distinct head, but the mouth parts which consist of the chelicerae and palps protrude beyond the anterior end of the body and are often spoken of erroneously as the 'head'. There are four pairs of legs, two pairs being situated towards

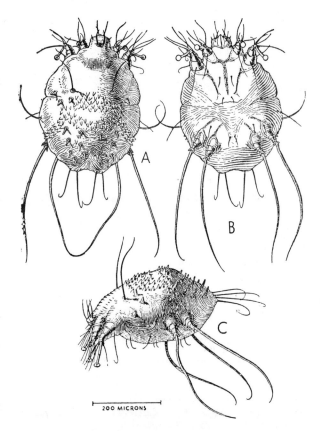

FIG. 1. Adult female of *Sarcoptes scabiei* de G. var *hominis*.

(a) Dorsal aspect.
(b) Ventral aspect.
(c) From the side.

the anterior and two towards the posterior end of the body. The basal joints of the legs are short and the anterior two pairs terminate in long unjointed stalks, bearing at their extremities distendable thin-walled sacs, usually spoken of as 'suckers'. The posterior two pairs of legs end in long bristles. The whole body of the mite is covered with characteristic grooves, and particularly on the dorsal side there is the elaborate arrangement of spines and bristles mentioned above. The internal structures with which the legs articulate (the epimeres) are scleratised and pigmented brown, and in a mounted specimen they are very clearly seen; in fact when *Sarcoptes* has been in Canada Balsam for a few weeks these epimeres are almost the only parts which have not become so transparent as to be practically invisible. The epimeres may be seen in Fig. 1*a* and in the male and larva in Fig. 2. The anus in *Sarcoptes* is situated terminally (this is a feature diagnostic of the genus ; many other acari have the anus in quite a different position). The eggs are laid through a slit about the middle of the ventral surface called the tocostome.

The adult male (Fig. 2*a*) is only about half as long as the female, but the difference in size appears to be due to the fact that the body of the female is much more distended (due to the enormous ovaries), while the hard parts (epimeres, etc.) are much the same size in the two sexes. Apart from size, the male differs from the female in its characteristic external genital apparatus, and because instead of having long bristles on the fourth pair of legs these appendages bear suckers attached by rather short stalks.

A word may be said here about these so-called 'suckers'. In most text-book drawings and in mounted preparations these organs appear exactly like rubber suckers. When, however, the *Sarcopies*

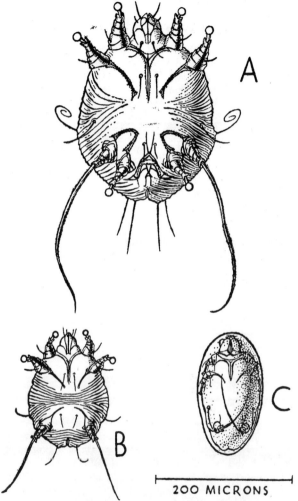

FIG. 2. Stages in the life history of *Sarcoptes*.

(a) Adult male.   (b) Larva.
(c) Egg containing developing embryo.

is examined alive a quite different appearance is
observed. The ' sucker ' is then seen to have no rigid
or definite shape, and tends to resemble a piece of
wet wash-leather on the end of a stick. The piece
of ' wet wash-leather ' is flapped down on to the
substratum, to which it may adhere quite firmly.
The typical sucker-like appearance is a post-mortem
effect. When mites are examined at temperatures
insufficient to stimulate activity, the appearance of
the suckers is one of the easiest ways of determining
whether an animal is alive or dead. In an immobilised
animal which is still alive the suckers are seldom
distended at all.

The other stages in the life-history of *Sarcoptes* are
the egg, the larva and the nymph. The egg (Fig. 2c) is
relatively enormous when compared with the size of
the adult. The egg figured here contains a fully
developed larva. The larva (Fig. 2b) is characterized
by possessing only three pairs of legs. The larva
moults and gives rise to the nymph ; this stage
possesses four pairs of legs. The nymph moults once
more, and then gives rise to either the adult male or
the immature female. The immature female is
approximately the same size as the male, and its
hard parts are the same size as those of the mature,
ovigerous individual. The transformation from
immature to ovigerous female probably occurs after
fertilisation, when the ovary swells up and distends
the body of the animal. In an ovigerous female the
ovary is responsible for more than half the internal
body contents, and variations in size of different
females are mainly due to whether or not there are
fully developed eggs inside this organ.

It is probable that the successful infection of a
new victim by *Sarcoptes* is usually accomplished by a
newly fertilized female. The mite is able to move
rapidly on the warm surface of the skin, traversing as

much as 2½ cm. (1 inch) in a minute. The parasite exercises some selection in the part of the body into which it burrows, the majority fixing on one of the normal ' sites of election ' (for details see Chapter II). The *Sarcoptes* takes approximately one hour to bury itself in the horny layer of the skin, and it never tunnels deeper than this. The statement common in text books that the mite can submerge itself in the cuticle in under three minutes is not borne out by careful observation of hundreds of mites. The process of burrowing is rather interesting. The legs and mouth parts are used to make the burrow. As well as ' biting ' its way into the skin with its jaws, the acarus uses the front two pairs of legs. The suckers adhere firmly to the surface and the animal gives the appearance of digging with its ' elbows ', *i.e.* there is a cutting edge on the last joint before the stalk which bears the suckers of each of the two front pairs of legs, and this is manipulated so as to tear through the layers of the epidermis.

The female mite usually remains in her burrow for the rest of her life. Occasionally, however, a newly-burrowed mite may leave her place in the epidermis a few hours after digging herself in, and wander over the skin until she finds a more suitable position. Once a mite has started a burrow properly she never leaves it of her own accord. Mites are frequently scratched out by the finger nails of their victims ; when this occurs many are killed, but a substantial proportion survive and burrow in again in another site. Sometimes a mite may be scratched out and transferred by the finger nails, but more often the scratching will remove the roof from the burrow and the parasite will walk away from this position. Only dead parasites have been discovered under the nails.

Within a few hours of starting her burrow the ovigerous female begins egg-laying. Two or three eggs are laid each day, and this process may go on for nearly two months. The eggs may be seen stuck to the floor of the burrow, and a biopsy made by cutting a whole burrow away in a thin slice of skin shows all its contents (Fig. 3). The female mite is visible at the anterior end, with the eggs all along the burrow behind her. In the preparation photographed in Fig. 3, 5 eggs, presumably laid within the last 2 days, lie immediately behind the mite ; no embryos are yet visible in these eggs. The next 2 eggs contain well-developed larvae. The remainder of the eggs (there are more than 20 in the preparation, only a few being included in the figure) have hatched, leaving only the empty shells behind. The small, black, oval-shaped objects in the burrow are the mite's faeces ; under the microscope they have an easily recognizable appearance. A preparation of this kind cannot reveal the total number of eggs which a female can lay, because the skin covering the older parts of a burrow gets worn away and the shells of the hatched eggs are lost. The speed at which the burrows are made is very variable, sometimes the animal progresses as much as 5 mm. a day, at other times she only moves about half a millimetre. Fig. 3 depicts a slowly-made burrow ; in it the eggs are close together. When the animal tunnels more rapidly (as in Fig. 6b) the eggs are scattered along the burrow. The speed at which the mite moves under the skin seems to have little influence on the rate of egg production.

The burrow is confined to the horny layer of the skin (see Fig. 4). The sites where the mites form burrows are not necessarily those in which the cuticle is thin, in fact regions with a thick cuticle are often attacked. In a position where the horny layer is fairly thick (i.e. ulna border of hand) the *Sarcoptes* forms its burrow within its depth ; in a thinner part

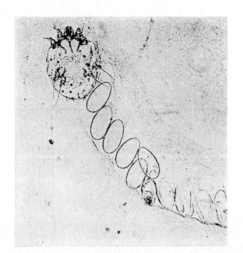

Fig 3. Whole mount of burrow of *Sarcoptes* containing adult female and eggs.

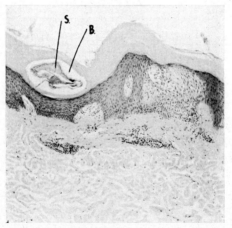

Fig. 4. Transverse section of skin showing burrow containing adult *Sarcoptes*.

S = *Sarcoptes*.   B = Lumen of burrow.

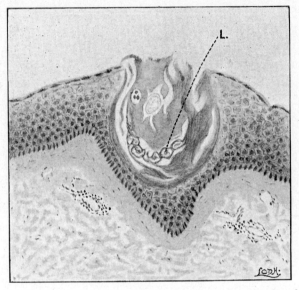

FIG. 5.   Transverse section of follicular papule containing larval
Sarcoptes.
L = Transverse section through legs and mouth parts of larva.

(*e.g.* on penis) the mite raises a tiny lump as it pushes aside the layers of the tissue.

The eggs take 3 or 4 days to hatch. It is often possible to find one or two larvae inside a burrow, but these have recently hatched for they always leave the burrows to continue their development. The idea that the immature *Sarcoptes* burrows into the tissues beneath the burrow is not supported by an examination of hundreds of burrows, and is probably a misconception caused by the study of other forms of acarine mange in animals. The larvae are able to move on the surface of the skin practically as rapidly as the adults, but they soon find shelter, and presumably also food, by entering hair follicles (Fig. 5). Both larvae and nymphs are to be found in hair follicles. As described above the nymphs moult to give rise to the adult male or the immature female ; this transformation occurs from 4 to 6 days after the hatching of the eggs. The adult males are not commonly found, and are undoubtedly much less common than the females, but whether this is due to a predominantly female sex-ratio or to a shorter life on the part of the males is not known for certain, but it is probable that the males do not live anything like as long as the females. The male *Sarcoptes* is found in a short burrow, less than a millimetre in length ; it probably remains inside this burrow for a short time only, and spends a considerable portion of its life on the skin surface in search of the unfertilized females. The unfertilized female likewise makes only a very small burrow, in which she may remain for a day or two only. Pairing probably occurs in the surface of the skin, and there is a very great mortality at this stage in development, for there must be a great deal of difficulty for the males and females, creatures only a fraction of a millimetre in length, to meet at all on the surface of the body of the scabies patient, whose skin surface will extend for several square metres.

The whole period of the life history from egg to ovigerous female may be as short as 10 days, but 14 days is a more normal period. There is in *Sarcoptes*, as in most parasitic forms of life, a considerable mortality during development, and it is often several weeks before the adult mites of the second generation make their appearance in a case of scabies. Well under 10 per cent. of the eggs ever give rise to adult mites.

It is a great advantage for anyone dealing with cases of scabies to be able to find and isolate the causative *Sarcoptes*. Once the parasite has been discovered, there is no shadow of doubt about the diagnosis. Undoubtedly any experienced dermatologist can diagnose the majority of cases of scabies without the need to search for acari, but for others without their experience the ability to find the parasite is the quickest short cut on the road to making an accurate diagnosis, and at present both army medical officers and physicians in civilian practice generally make at least a 25 per cent. error in their diagnosis of scabies. In the next chapter some details regarding the parts of the body most commonly attacked by *Sarcoptes* are given ; here I propose to give some details of how I have found it easiest to isolate the parasites. The ovigerous female is the stage most easily found, and to remove the animal it is essential to know just what to look for. I have seen many medical officers trying to follow text-book instructions, blindly sticking, cutting, and scraping the skin and looking at every bit of debris under the microscope ; it is not surprising that their search is so rarely successful. The first preliminary to finding the *Sarcoptes* is to discover an inhabited burrow and to observe the position of the animal. Fig. 6*a* is a magnified surface

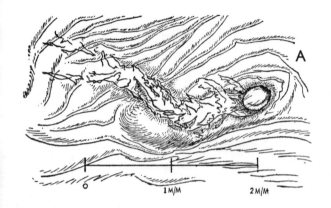

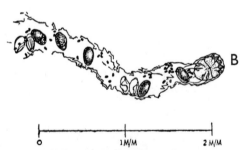

FIG. 6.   The burrow of *Sarcoptes*.

(a) Enlarged surface drawing.
(b) Whole mount of biopsy of same burrow.

view of such a burrow. The mite is visible at the anterior end as a raised whitish oval with dark pigmentation at its front. This pigmentation is caused by the appearance of the epimeres connected with the mouth parts and anterior limbs. The burrow of Fig. 6a was removed in a thin slice of skin, cut off parallel to the body surface with a safety razor blade and then mounted in Berlese's fluid,[1] a liquid which fixes, clears, and makes a permanent preparation of the tissues. This type of biopsy is a simple one for making mounts to show the contents of burrows, but once the mite has been seen through the surface layer of the skin the simplest procedure is merely to take an ordinary needle mounted in a wooden handle and reflex the skin covering the animal. After this a little ' fishing about ' will generally result in finding the Sarcoptes stuck to the needle, or sometimes after this disturbance it may walk out of the now uncovered trench on to the surface of the skin. Dead and live mites stick equally readily to a needle, so the animals cannot be holding on as is often alleged. This process can be done with the naked eye, but some magnification is an aid ; a watchmaker's lens gives a convenient magnification and leaves the hands free. It cannot be too strongly urged that the whole secret of finding the Sarcoptes is to know what to look for and not to try to hunt blindly over the body surface.

If the operator is used to removing mites, there is little doubt when the animal is adhering to the needle, but to make certain that it is indeed a Sarcoptes a magnification of 50 diametres is quite sufficient. Dermatologists usually place the acarus in liquor potassae on a slide and cover with a cover-slip. In my opinion it is more satisfactory to place the animal on to a clean slide and examine it without any clearing medium at all. In cool weather the slide can then be

[1] For formula see Appendix.

warmed and if the mite has not been damaged it will walk in its characteristic manner. Most patients are very interested to see a living acarus under the microscope, and after such a demonstration it is easier to secure their wholehearted co-operation in ensuring thorough treatment.

CHAPTER II

THE PARASITOLOGY OF HUMAN SCABIES

MANY common misconceptions exist concerning the number of parasites found in patients suffering from scabies, for it is generally believed that there are thousands of itch mites present in every case. This is quite untrue and the small number of parasites actually present explains the difficulty which competent medical officers have in detecting any parasites at all in the majority of their patients. Nevertheless, if one knows where to look and what to look for, it should be possible by careful examination to find parasites in every case of active scabies ; if it is not possible to find mites, then active scabies can be excluded, though the time and skill required to be sure that one can exclude *Sarcoptic* infection is much greater than that required to make the positive diagnosis.

In this chapter a brief account of the range of numbers of parasites found on a random selection of scabies patients will be given. Actually only adult female *Sarcoptes* have been accurately enumerated, but as these probably bear a definite relation to the total mite population an estimation of this stage alone should serve as a reasonable guide to the size of the total population. For convenience, the number of adult females will be referred to as the ' parasite rate '. The total number of other stages, including eggs, larvae, nymphs, and immature females, may possibly be twenty times as great as the parasite rate, but experimental work suggests that some considerable part of the very great mortality which takes place

14

during development will eliminate a large proportion of all these stages.

Fig. 7 gives some data concerning the parasite rate found from examinations made of nearly 900 adult male patients. The mean parasite rate was 11·3 ; more than half the patients had between 1

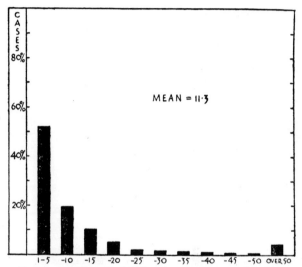

FIG. 7. Numbers of adult female mites in cases of scabies.

and 5 adult female *Sarcoptes* and only some 3 per cent. had over 50. The greatest parasite rate discovered was 511. It is at first sight very remarkable that such small numbers as these should be responsible for the widespread signs and symptoms of clinical scabies. Some explanation of the facts concerned is given in the next chapter. Incidentally, the extremely small parasite rate in human scabies is vastly different from what is found in sarcoptic mange in animals, where many thousands of parasites may occur on a single host. Norwegian or crusted scabies in man would appear to simulate the condition found in animals ; no case of this form of the disease has been reported in Britain in recent years.

The intensity of parasitic infection at the time when patients are received for treatment bears no direct relation to the intensity of discomfort experienced by the victim. Some of those cases with

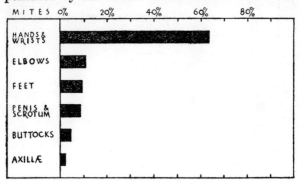

FIG. 8.   Sites of adult female mites in cases of scabies.

very small parasite rates complained of intolerable itching, and others with a much larger number of acari appeared to suffer little inconvenience.

It is well known that certain parts of the body harbour mites more than others, and an analysis of the distribution of the adult females is given in Fig. 8. This diagram is based on the same cases as were used to demonstrate the parasite rate. The majority (63 per cent.) of the mites were found on the hands and wrists ; the next most favoured site was the extensor aspect of the elbows, where 10·9 per

cent. of the acari occurred. The feet and genitals
had about 9 per cent. each, the buttocks 4 per cent.,
the axillae 2 per cent., and on the whole remaining
surface of the body only 2 per cent. of the mite
population.

If patients have to be examined rapidly it may
not always be possible to examine all the different
parts of the body, so that it is of value to know which
sites are most likely to be invaded by *Sarcoptes*. Of
the almost 900 cases considered earlier in this chapter,
85 per cent. had one or more mites on the hands and
wrists and an examination of the arms alone would
have made possible a certain diagnosis in 9 cases out
of 10. Whenever possible, if large numbers of individuals have to be examined to exclude scabies, the
whole of the skin surface should be examined, but
when this is impossible (as for instance in routine
school inspections) it is perhaps reassuring to realize
that the majority of cases could be detected by a
properly carried out scrutiny of selected areas of the
body.

Those familiar with clinical scabies may be surprised
at these results, which show that more than 60 per
cent. of the mites are likely to occur on the hands
and wrists, while comparatively small numbers will
be found on the genitals and buttocks. The more
commonly held view is that, particularly in soldiers,
the hands are rarely affected and the genitals and
buttocks are the regions most commonly attacked.
This discrepancy may be explained by a study of the
reactions of the various parts of the body to attack by
Sarcoptes. The hands and wrists give comparatively
little reaction as compared with the softer parts of
the body. The intense reactions set up, for instance,
on the genitals and buttocks, stimulate the patient to
scratch ; scratching causes the obvious signs by which
scabies is often diagnosed, but it also frequently

destroys the mites. Lesions on the genitals, which occur on nearly every male patient, show that infestation of this region has taken place in the past, but nine times out of ten the invading acari are destroyed by the nails of their victims. Ecthymatous areas on the buttocks are also exceedingly common. In this region irritation may be caused by mites, or as part of a general sensitization (see Chapter III), and whatever the cause, scratching occurs. The buttocks are particularly liable to bacterial infection of lesions caused by scratching, and this will give rise to obvious stigmata. Also it will exterminate any mites if they are present and have not been scratched out.

The distribution of the parasites in children and adult females has not been so fully investigated. In babies burrows can occur on all parts of the body, including the face, the palms of the hands and the soles of the feet. The largest number of mites appears to occur on the feet during the first year of life, and it is probably not until about the fifth year that the hands and wrists come to bear the majority of the population. In women the nipples are said to form one of the most frequently infected sites.

One might expect that if a case of scabies were not treated the parasite rate would go on increasing for a very long period. A study of what happened in a dozen infected volunteers who went for up to nine months without treatment reveals that this is not the case. The parasite rate in these volunteers always increased during the first two or three months of the first infection suffered by each patient, and at the end of that period a parasite rate varying in different individuals between about 20 and about 400 was produced ; the maximum value depended on various factors, some of which are discussed in later chapters. After the mites reached the values just mentioned there was either no more increase or actually a fall in numbers. There was considerable individual variation, some of the patients showing a rapid fall in parasitic rate until a complete and spontaneous cure resulted. Others decreased their parasites to very small numbers, but remained infected till the end of the period. The remainder showed considerable fluctuations in parasite rate, the numbers of inhabited burrows decreasing and increasing in an irregular manner. Incidentally it may be repeated that no matter how rapidly the population increased, it never passed 10 per cent. of the potential increase which the egg production of the females might have led us to expect. This means that there was always a wastage of at least 90 per cent.

Eggs and immature stages of *Sarcoptes*, though difficult to find, are probably much more numerous than ovigerous females. As the larvae and nymphs wander about the body surface during part of their existence it is obvious that they are likely to be transferred from one person to another. Nevertheless it is probably very uncommon for these immature stages alone to give rise to a permanent infection. A burrowing ovigerous female gives rise to a continual stream of immature stages, and though there is such a great mortality yet the chances are that in time some of the acari will complete their life history successfully, be fertilized and begin new burrows. If even quite a large number of larvae or nymphs is picked up, though there is a chance that one or more successful burrows will be established, it is more likely that the mites will all die out. When all the ovigerous females are removed from a normal case of human scabies (with ten or less inhabited burrows) in the majority of cases the disease dies out without further treatment, though there must have been left a considerable number of immature stages of *Sarcoptes*.

Removal of the adult acari from more heavily infected cases does not cure the disease, so that there is a limit to the number of immature stages which can safely be left, but the chance of picking up anything like this number is a very remote one. Direct experiments attempting to infect with eggs and immature mites have only succeeded in producing crops of papules and no permanent infections.

The information given in this and the preceding chapter will, it is hoped, make it possible for the reader, after a little practical experience with cases of scabies, to find and remove acari without difficulty. The first essential is to know what to look for (see Fig. 6a) ; the second is to know where to look (see Fig. 8).

CHAPTER III

THE DEVELOPMENT OF SYMPTOMS

In a typical case of scabies diagnosis is not difficult. The patient complains of severe itching which becomes intolerable at night, often keeping him awake. An examination of the body reveals a characteristic rash. This rash is in part due to the parasites, but to a greater extent it is caused by the patient scratching himself. Most patients show, even at a distance, erythematous patches and follicular papules in the areas shown in Fig. 9. If a patient has a history of itching, worst at night, and a characteristic rash, then it is advisable to suspect scabies. The diagnosis can, however, only be made certain by the discovery of burrows and if possible the isolation of the parasite. A description of the simplest procedure for finding parasites is given above in Chapter I. Not uncommonly cases of scabies do not present a completely typical appearance and it is here that the ability to find the parasites is of real value, for if every doubtful case is treated as scabies the parasiticidal substance used, which is in itself likely to be a skin irritant, may cause severe dermatitis in sensitive conditions which are sometimes confused with scabies. Furthermore, efficient methods of treatment sometimes get an unwarranted bad name as they fail to clear up conditions wrongly disgnosed as scabies.

Most text books of dermatology show excellent photographs of scabietic patients. Actually these figures depict mainly the results of secondary infection following primary scabies, as it is almost impossible to produce a satisfactory photograph of simple, uncomplicated scabies.

3

It has generally been thought that the itching in scabies is caused by the active movements of the burrowing mites and because the itching tends to be worse at night this has made people think that the

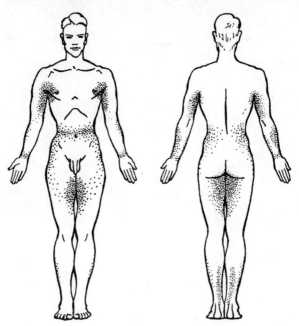

Fig. 9.   Scabies "rash."   (Note: the rash does *not* correspond with the sites of election of the acari.)

mites are mainly nocturnal in their activity.   Actually it is possible for people to have mites burrowing actively in their cuticle for weeks, without causing the least sensation.   Not only is this possible, but it is apparently a universal occurrence at certain stages of every person's infection with scabies. If even a considerable number of mites tunnel into the cuticle of a person who has never had scabies before, although typical burrows will be visible if they are looked for carefully with a lens, no typical lesions and no generalized papular rash will be visible. The patient will probably notice no symptoms of itching whatever. After a period of roughly a month, though apparently in some individuals this period may be considerably prolonged, a complete change occurs. Erythematous patches appear around the burrows and rings of follicular papules several inches wide become apparent in this vicinity. It is at this stage that itching starts and further signs, caused by the scratching which the itching promotes, will also begin to appear. The extent to which these signs are widespread will depend to some extent on the mite population which has been built up in the non-sensitive or incubation period.

I believe that in scabies a true sensitization occurs. A similar process has been described in connexion with the bites of certain insects which attack man. Some individuals, for instance, when first bitten by a new species of mosquito, give no skin reaction, but when the bites are repeated a few weeks later swelling and irritation are noticed at once. In the same way as an insect bite itches long after the insect has departed, so the lesions caused by *Sarcoptes* may remain irritant although no parasite has occupied them for quite a long period. This gives further proof that the itching is not caused by the activity of the parasite.

In a sensitized individual it is not uncommon to find vesicles as large as grains of wheat underlying the burrows (the edge of such a vesicle in the deeper layers of the epidermis can be seen to the right of Fig. 4). The vesicles are a few millimetres behind the mites, for though the parasites are responsible for their occurrence it takes the tissues some 24 hours to react and in this period the animals have progressed further. Scratching will often rupture the vesicles and they then form foci of sepsis following bacterial invasion.

Particularly in small children one frequently gets crops of small vesicles, quite apart from those connected with burrows. These vesicles occur particularly on the hands and feet ; they often persist for weeks after efficient treatment, and make it difficult to distinguish between cured and uncured cases.

The skin sensations felt in scabies are quite complicated and volunteers who have been infected with the disease describe several distinct reactions. As mentioned above, practically nothing is felt during the first month or so of a primary infection. A slight intermittent itching around the positions where the burrows exist is sometimes described, but as this is not accompanied by erythema and as the volunteer has known that a burrow exists it is possible that the itching is mainly due to imagination. Once sensitization has occurred a variety of different sensations are experienced, and the description given here summarizes the experiences of a number of individuals, although these volunteers have disagreed on certain minor points. The burrow of the adult female gave a characteristic sensation which is described as ' intermittent ' and starting suddenly with an almost biting intensity. The feeling has been described as ' not unpleasant ' and there is no doubt that it was distinguishable from other feelings because volunteers have been able to locate, accurately, new burrows before these had actually been observed. With a man who had had some experience of the disease, nine times out of ten, if he suggested there was a new burrow in a certain region it was possible to discover it by careful examination. Certain areas of the body become covered with follicular papules, probably due to the activity of the immature stages. The areas covered with these papules were irritated but the feeling was quite distinct from that caused by the burrows. This more or less localized ' papule itching ' was said by some to differ from the generalized sensitization which took place, and affected the abdomen, thighs, and other areas in which there was little evidence of actual parasitic invasion. Secondarily infected areas were sometimes devoid of sensation, but were also inclined to itch in a manner which is generally described as ' unpleasant.' After the patient was cured the itching sensations by no means always disappeared. Several individuals have reported that the sites of the old burrows itch intermittently, giving feelings very similar to those experienced when the living parasites were there. The generalized skin sensitization also persisted in certain cases.

Severe itching which accompanies scabies is then due to a sensitization of the host and until this sensitization occurs diagnosis is practically impossible. This long period of incubation has been observed in about fifty volunteers infected on known dates, but the same conclusion has been confirmed by clinical workers. In fever hospitals patients who are admitted apparently entirely free from scabies and who are kept under conditions of strict isolation, frequently develop symptoms of the disease many weeks after their admission. At the beginning of the present war, in reception areas, it was not infrequently found that evacuee children developed scabies some time after arriving at their new billets. The medical authorities from evacuation areas were frequently blamed for sending out children without proper preliminary examination. This undoubtedly did occur, but it is probable that some of the evacuees were incubating scabies, though at the time of their evacuation there were no symptoms and diagnosis was practically impossible. A similar state of affairs is said to have occurred at the end of the last war, when men were demobilized or posted from one locality to another ; they set out apparently free from scabies but developed symptoms at a later date.

Some patients with fairly obvious scabies insist that symptoms of itching are completely absent. Some of them have obviously scratched themselves severely and it is likely that they come from those sections of the population in which, if a person itches, he subconsciously scratches the offending area and relieves the sensation, without any thought of scratching and without any fear of offending his social code. There are also, however, occasional individuals who show all the other signs of sensitivity (erythema round the burrows, follicular papules, etc.) without any noticeable scratch marks, so it is possible that itching is not a universal symptom even of advanced scabies.

When a patient who has had scabies once, and has therefore become sensitized, is reinfected, he gives an entirely different picture from that found in a person who has never had the disease before. Within perhaps only a few hours the sites where mites are burrowing (there is actually usually only one) become inflamed and a considerable irritation is felt. Under these conditions it is not infrequent for the invading parasite to be scratched out and the infection stopped. In this way a curious sort of immunity is produced in some individuals. Further, the oedema which surrounds the burrows in a sensitized person may render the cuticle unpalatable and may cause the mite to vacate its burrow voluntarily. The already sensitized individual may sometimes give rise to general symptoms more rapidly than the patient developing the disease for the first time, but more often sensitization is a sort of protective reaction, and although local symptoms may develop soon, the way in which the parasites are kept down by scratching is sufficient to prevent the development of a mite population large enough to cause general cutaneous symptoms. The only exception is when a sensitized person is being constantly reinfected with numerous parasites, as when he sleeps, night after night, together with someone with a large parasite population. He may then develop general symptoms in a week or so.

Incidentally, if patients become sensitized to *Sarcoptes*, so that they give the considerable reaction referred to above, it might be expected, on analogy with other instances of a similar sort, that at least some cases would eventually become immune and would then tolerate the parasites without further reaction. I have not seen any direct evidence of this, but it is possible that in Norwegian scabies we have such cases and the symptoms there are the direct consequence of the huge numbers of parasites in a host which does not itch or scratch.

It is not easy to discover exactly why burrows are commoner in certain sites than in others. The adult female *Sarcoptes* does appear to exercise some selection and mites liberated on the bodies of volunteers frequently find their way to the normal sites of election. Further, mites which are compelled to burrow in the uncharacteristic areas may voluntarily come out of the pockets in the cuticle, into which they have submerged themselves, and make their way to a more favoured spot. In addition to the selective powers of the parasite, the reactions of the host influence the positions of burrows. The normal sites of election are, to some extent, areas where the least reaction is given by the skin and so there is the least tendency for the parasites to be scratched out. It is perhaps noteworthy that during the first part of their primary infection volunteers appear to be more prone to develop burrows on uncharacteristic sites. After the patients become sensitized it is likely that any mites which started to burrow in such an area would give an instant reaction and be removed by the finger nails.

In the war of 1914–18 it was not uncommon to find soldiers suffering from scabies and body lice. Under these conditions unless burrows were carefully sought the scabies infection was very frequently overlooked, as the signs of scabies were often masked by those of pediculosis.

Certain other symptoms have been connected with scabies; for instance, albuminuria has been said to have occurred commonly. We have tested the urine of several hundred cases of scabies and on two occasions only traces of albumen have been found, and no case of serious albuminuria has been detected. This is true both of simple scabies and of cases complicated by pustular secondary infection. Eosinophilia is also said to occur commonly in scabies. An examination of both lightly and heavily infected persons does not support this contention.

CHAPTER IV

SECONDARY PATHOLOGICAL CONDITIONS INDUCED BY SCABIES INFECTION

THE simple parasitic infection of scabies may be a comparatively trivial matter. In its early stages it causes no distressing symptoms. Later, inflammation and pruritis occur, but if the disease is diagnosed at this stage treatment is simple and a complete cure should be rapidly obtained. Unfortunately a distressingly high proportion of cases is not diagnosed until a more serious condition has arisen and secondary infection has set in.

The vast majority of people who develop scabies do not seek medical attention at all, at any rate until some severe disability has affected them or some near connexion of theirs. If the itching is very troublesome they may consult their local chemist (drug store); with scabies, as with other diseases, far more people go for free advice to a chemist than to a doctor. Fortunately large numbers of chemists readily recognize scabies and either prescribe an efficient medicament or advise the patient to seek medical attention. Frequently, however, no one is consulted and the choice of medicament depends on the whim of the patient and the advertisements he has read in his Sunday newspaper. In my experience the majority of people who develop scabies buy a widely advertised specific 'for all skin diseases'; fortunately this is quite innocuous and hardly ever causes a serious dermatitis, but on the other hand it has no effect on *Sarcoptes*. The more unfortunate patient buys an effective remedy like sulphur ointment, but as this is applied without proper supervision incomplete cures, combined with severe treatment dermatitis are the usual results.

A scabies infection receiving no treatment at all (and here we may include scabies treated with most widely advertised patent medicines and ointments) may end in three different ways, which are as follows :

(1) By constant scratching the patient may eventually destroy all the parasites and cure himself. If he has been using some innocuous medicament he may give it the credit for his recovery, although he would probably have recovered as rapidly anyhow.

(2) Although the patient does not obtain a complete cure, he will reduce the number of parasites to very small proportions, but he may continue for years with a low grade infection. He will always itch and scratch but will get so used to these reactions that he will hardly be incommoded by the presence of the parasites.

(3) In the more serious cases, which we are now considering, the constant scratching damages the skin which then becomes infected by other organisms. Pustules, boils, ecthymata, impetigo or eczema result, and the patient may be so seriously affected that prolonged hospital treatment is necessary.

One early result of sensitization in scabies is the production of follicular papules on various parts of the body. Scratching will frequently cause these papules to be invaded by bacteria and transformed into pustules ; more or less widespread pustules of this kind form the commonest sort of secondary infection. Quite commonly, in addition to ordinary pustules, boils also appear. The main trouble with an infection which takes the form of pustules and boils is that this secondary condition is very apt to persist for a very long time after the primary infection of *Sarcoptes* has been eliminated.

Impetigo contagiosa is a common accompaniment of scabies, particularly in children. In the first instance the impetigo tends to affect the scabietic lesions on the various parts of the body, but later the infection is generally transmitted to the face. As scabies is known not to affect the face, except in babies, a secondary impetigo in this region often causes the scabies to be overlooked.

A fair proportion of cases of neglected scabies give rise to ecthyma. The buttocks and legs are the regions most commonly affected, and sometimes very extensive ecthyma will be found in patients on whom practically no parasites can be discovered. It is useless trying to find *Sarcoptes* in the middle of an area of ecthyma, for the pus will have exterminated the acari, though it is sometimes possible to find a few mites in the areas of healthy skin at the borders of the ecthymatous areas.

Why some cases of scabies develop extensive secondary infection while others are not so affected is not fully understood. Bodily cleanliness is of some importance, for in a dirty skin there are likely to be far more micro-organisms to invade the abraded skin. It may be pointed out that we know very little concerning the reasons why some individuals are more likely than others to develop boils and such-like skin infections ; individuals liable to these complaints will perhaps be most liable to develop secondary infections following on scabies. The general health of the patient is of importance and secondary infections will be more likely to develop in a person whose vitality is impaired than in a more resistant subject. Diet is probably of importance and a population suffering from malnutrition may be expected to be particularly prone to develop secondary infection following scabies. Much more research is required on these problems but they should be tackled not only as they concern scabies but in connexion with the whole question of skin infection.

Eczema develops not infrequently in cases of long-standing scabies. In individuals who are susceptible to eczema, the added stimulus to the skin caused by the *Sarcoptes* will frequently be sufficient to precipitate a further attack. The eczematous rash may tend to mask the scabies, but a distribution resembling that of the generalized rash shown in Fig. 9 should make one suspect that scabies is the underlying cause. Even after the scabies has been successfully treated the eczema may persist for a long time ; it is important to avoid over-treatment of the scabies as the medicaments used are such as are likely to make an existing eczema considerably worse.

No simple rules can be set down for the treatment of the different kinds of secondary infection. I believe that it is always advisable to treat the scabies, which is the primary cause of the trouble, first ; in this way it is possible that the itching may be diminished and the patient will thus be less inclined to scratch and to spread the secondary infection. This view is not universally held, and some workers prefer to clean up impetigo before tackling scabies, particularly in children, where acaricidal medicaments may be painful if there are many unhealed sores.

In severe pustular scabies, where the burrows have been transformed into lacunae of pus, itching may be almost entirely absent. This is probably due to the fact that *Sarcoptes* cannot survive in pus and many cases described as severe pustular scabies may have no remaining itch mites alive on their bodies. The sensations caused by these pustular lesions differ greatly in different individuals; some volunteers have stated that secondarily infected areas in scabies can be distinguished by a quite distinct and rather painful feeling.

Itching is the principal symptom of scabies, and one trouble is that in a proportion of cases the itching continues for a long time after the scabies has been cured. It is exceedingly difficult to distinguish such a case from the result of insufficient treatment; the only really satisfactory method is by the discovery or otherwise of living *Sarcoptes*. If living adult mites cannot be found, but an area of follicular papules is observed around a region where it is believed that an active burrow may exist, it is not improbable that the parasitic infection may persist.

In this question of persistent itching, psychological factors may play an important part. If the patient believes that he has been cured he will, for a few days after treatment, be less troubled by itching than another who thinks that his treatment has been inefficient; this is still true if the former is treated with a substance that has practically no acaricidal properties and the latter with a medicament which is 100 per cent. efficient. There is generally more trouble in treating patients who are worried or ashamed because they have caught scabies than in treating those who take such an ailment as a matter of course. The worried patient magnifies the importance of the least residual itch and often resorts to further self-treatment with a resultant dermatitis. Others who think that there is something 'dirty' about scabies will resort to taking several baths a day, probably all accompanied by vigorous scrubbing; this may eventually produce an eczematization of the skin.

It has been said that over-treatment of scabies leads to more serious trouble than the disease itself. This is sometimes true and it occurs not only among people who treat themselves, but among those who are under medical supervision. The question of the treatment of scabies is dealt with in detail in a later chapter, and it need only be said here that if sulphur ointment is used, three proper applications are the most that should ever be used in one course of treatment, and a complete cure will usually be obtained with less. More than three inunctions is very likely to give a serious dermatitis ; the worst case I have seen was a child under medical supervision who had used the ointment daily for *five months* ! Over-treatment with benzyl benzoate preparations will also give a dermatitis, though the emulsion in water is less dangerous than most other medicaments.

The frequent routine inspections of members of the Services in this country have the result that scabies is usually detected at a fairly early stage, before much secondary infection has arisen. The only exception is in the case of new recruits, and when men are suffering from the after-effects of some unsatisfactory method of treatment (*e.g.* Thiosulphate and HCl) . . . fortunately these latter are now very rare. Civilians on the whole are not subject to routine inspections and it is among them that serious secondary infection arises, particularly in pre-school age children. During the last war, however, a very different state of affairs existed, for men with scabies under conditions of poor hygiene inseparable from trench warfare often developed very grave secondary infection. If the comparatively trivial parasitic infection which many of them must have had before they entered the trenches had been diagnosed, much suffering and loss of man-power would have been avoided. All troubles concerning secondary infection would be avoided if one could guarantee 100 per cent. early diagnosis ; this is only possible when the medical officers concerned are thoroughly familiar with *Sarcoptes*.

CHAPTER V

THE TRANSMISSION OF SCABIES

THERE has been a great deal of controversy concerning the way in which scabies is transmitted. Very divergent views are held concerning the ease with which the disease can be transmitted or picked up. It has sometimes been suggested that anyone suffering from scabies is a grave danger if he travels in public conveyances or even mixes in the street with his fellow-citizens. The opposite view is also held and it is suggested that if an adult contracts scabies it is his own fault and through circumstances entirely under his own control. Much argument has concerned the importance or otherwise of fomites, particularly bedding and blankets. Some investigators have considered that these are of no importance in the transmission of scabies while others have blamed such apparently unlikely things as canvas sheets from under mattresses and the straw from inside palliasses.

Scabies is essentially a domestic disease. There is no evidence that under present conditions it is frequently transmitted from soldier to soldier during the course of his normal military duties. Cases of scabies in the Army are sporadic and I have certainly never seen anything to suggest that a whole batch from one tent or house have infected one another. A similar state of affairs is found in schools. Though scabies is distressingly common among school children there is no evidence to show that transmission occurs inside the school-room. A few children from all parts of the school will generally be found to be infected and more often than not the children concerned will all be found to be members of one or two families. A certain amount of transmission may take place in overcrowded air-raid shelters, but there is little evidence to suggest that scabies is frequently transmitted in those places. The incidence of the disease has increased as much in the cities which have not been bombed, and in which no one lives in communal shelters, as in those other cities with large air-raid shelter populations.

During the last war it is probable that on active service, when men were living in crowded dug-outs, a certain amount of scabies transmission took place. Some transmission of the disease occurs in lunatic asylums and in hostels occupied by large numbers of evacuees.

There has been a certain amount of experimental work on the transmission of the disease. Non-infected volunteers have been subjected to various conditions which might be thought to be liable to give rise to infection. A comparison has been made of the results of treatment and of the relapse rate when all fomites have been sterilized, and when no fomites have received any attention. These experiments have given some indication of the ways in which scabies is most likely to be transmitted.

Bedding is certainly able to transmit scabies. If a bed is slept in by a scabies patient one night, and then the next night it is occupied by some other person there is a risk that the latter will contract the disease. This risk, however, is an exceedingly small one, and probably the chances are less than 1 in 200 that scabies will be picked up. If this is true for a bed which it is known has been used by a scabies patient, then the risks of transmission from casual beds or from inefficiently laundered bedding must be exceedingly remote. In certain circumstances however they cannot be entirely ignored.

Communal towels, particularly in schools, have

4

often been blamed for transmitting scabies. I do not think that these are of much importance. In some experiments towels have been used by many hundreds of cases of scabies and later used again by uninfected volunteers without a single instance of transmission.

In addition to blaming bedding and towels, many other inanimate objects have been accused of spreading scabies. Money, seats and straps in public conveyances, chairs and tables in clubs, baths, and last but not least, lavatory seats, have all been blamed for the spread of scabies. I believe that none of these are of major importance. When, under carefully controlled conditions, infected and uninfected volunteers lived together for many months in the same house, using all the same facilities and conveniences, no cases of infection appeared in the ' control ' group of people. At least, among adults the ordinary social contacts are unlikely to spread scabies.

In distinction to the difficulty of transmitting scabies by the intermediary of an inanimate object, personal contact, particularly of a prolonged nature, spreads the disease very readily. The most certain way of contracting the disease is to sleep in a bed together with somebody suffering from scabies. In this connexion it should be remembered that it may take two months for symptoms to develop and that during at least the latter part of this period the person who is developing the disease will be quite as infective as another person showing all the classical symptoms. Again, this long period which the disease may take to develop makes it very difficult to trace the contacts of cases which are seen in a well developed stage.

Among soldiers and other young adult males a high proportion of cases of scabies is contracted in a venereal manner, though it is probably more frequent for a married man to become infected when at home on leave than for infection to take place during illicit intercourse. Under these latter conditions contact may be of a briefer nature and scabies is more a disease transmitted by sleeping together than actually by sexual intercourse. There seems to be little doubt that children are frequently the first members of a house to be infected and they probably sometimes transmit infection to each other through holding hands or playing in various ways. Pastimes such as dancing or ' petting ' in cinemas, which allow prolonged skin-to-skin contact under conditions warm enough to make the *Sarcoptes* thoroughly motile, will no doubt encourage transmission.

The site of lesions on the body of a patient gives little in the way of a satisfactory clue to the site of original infection. *Sarcoptes* can move so rapidly on the surface of the skin that even although it is picked up on one part of the body it may easily walk to another before settling to burrow. I have seen it stated that the presence of patches of ecthymatous impetigo on the buttocks suggests that lavatory seats are a likely source of infection. This is not necessarily the case and it should particularly be noted that although this ecthymatous condition occurs very frequently very few mites are actually found in the region of the buttocks. The buttocks forms one of the areas where itching is particularly intense, even though no parasites are there and bacterial infection of any scratch marks is particularly likely.

As mentioned in an earlier chapter, conditions which are responsible for the rapid development of secondary infection may sometimes be wrongly blamed for the transmission of scabies. I think, for instance, in the last war, men in the trenches may have transmitted scabies among themselves to a limited extent, but more commonly it was secondary pyodermic infections which were rampant and which were particularly prone to develop to an acute stage in persons already suffering from scabies.

It has been the usual process to disinfest as many as possible of the possessions of a scabies patient in order to prevent reinfection. There is a considerable amount of doubt as to whether this is really necessary. Hebra, in the middle of last century, found he got less than 5 per cent. of recurrences when no sterilization at all was practised. I myself have treated many cases without sterilizing blankets or clothing, without getting any substantial number of recurrences. The main advantage of sterilization is that it makes the patient feel that something serious is being done and gives him more confidence in the treatment. Most areas where sterilization is regularly carried out have also efficient facilities for treatment of the patients themselves, and any comparison of the results in two different areas employing different methods is very difficult to interpret. At present the general consensus of opinion appears to be that if facilities are easily obtainable sterilization should be practised, but the risks of reinfection from not sterilizing clothing and bedding are considerably smaller than those from overlooking cases of latent infection.

A study of the biology of the *Sarcoptes* throws some light on the processes of transmission. It also reveals how sterilization should be carried out if such a process is deemed worth while. The mite is unable to withstand a high temperature and dies within 10 minutes at 50° C. (120° F.). The moisture contained in the air makes no difference to this thermal death point. It should be remembered that in any disinfestor it may be difficult to ensure that the necessary temperature is reached by all the innermost clothes or blankets, and that if moist materials are disinfested using dry heat, evaporation may reduce the temperature at the surface of the cloth and so prevent proper sterilization taking place.

If no proper sterilization apparatus exists, and if it is believed that, without disinfesting, fomites are a serious risk in spreading the disease, then, as *Sarcoptes* can only live for a short time away from man it is valuable to know how long bedding, etc., should be stored to ensure that none of the parasites could possibly survive. *Sarcoptes* lives longest at about 13° C. (55° F.) when the air is moist, but even under these conditions none will live for as long as a fortnight. Under conditions found in a drying cupboard it is unlikely that any itch mites will survive longer than 2 days. The ordinary processes of laundering should be sufficient to exterminate the parasite.

Sarcoptes is a creature which is adapted to living in or on the skin of man, where it will normally experience only a very narrow range of temperature. The animal appears to have no organs for appreciating light and its behaviour is not influenced in any way by the intensity or direction of illumination. *Sarcoptes* is completely immobilized by the ordinary sort of temperatures which are found in rooms in Britain in winter. Below 16° C. (61° F.) the animal is in complete chill coma and even up to 20° C. (68° F.) practically no movement takes place. It would thus be impossible for the animal to walk, for instance, from one bed to another in an unheated bedroom, though when warm skin from one individual comes in contact with that of another transmission should be able to take place readily.

When *Sarcoptes* is exposed to a temperature gradient it is found never to move to the colder parts of the range. Its behaviour is such that if it strays from the skin on to the cooler clothing or bedding, it is more likely to find its way back to the skin than it is to wander farther afield.

The behaviour and biology of the mite is therefore such that it appears unlikely that large numbers (and usually only small numbers are present on the body) will migrate on to clothing or blankets. For this reason sterilization may often be dispensed with. If, however, sterilization is considered necessary, comparatively low temperatures will easily kill all stages of the parasite. It should be remembered that the more intimate garments are those most likely to transmit the disease or perhaps to cause a reinfection of a treated person. As however, most treatments cover the patient with a layer of an acaricidal substance, if infected clothing is replaced while the substance is still on the skin this alone may serve as an efficient method of sterilization. Sufficient benzyl benzoate remains on the skin for at least 12 hours to kill *Sarcoptes* on the inner garments.

In Chapter II it is shown that about 3 per cent. of cases of scabies have very large populations of parasites. These few highly parasitized individuals may be of overwhelming importance in the epidemiology of the disease, for they may cause transmission under circumstances where the ordinary lightly infected case would not.

After reviewing the most recent work, the Advisory Committee on Scabies of the Ministry of Health have recommended that the disinfestation of the clothing and blankets of scabies patients may reasonably be dispensed with.

CHAPTER VI

THE INCIDENCE OF SCABIES

THERE seems no doubt that the incidence of scabies varies greatly from time to time, but it is very difficult to obtain any accurate information concerning the proportion of the population suffering from the disease. Scabies is not notifiable, so no general records of cases are kept (see, however, footnote on p. 52). Even when some attempt has been made to keep an account of the cases of scabies in a district, as there is often an error in the diagnosis of at least 25 per cent. it is difficult to assess the value of the results.

War is commonly believed to be the usual cause of an epidemic of scabies and Friedman in his book *Scabies, Civil and Military* has gone to considerable lengths to correlate all recent scabies epidemics with outbreaks of hostilities. He gives detailed accounts of all existing data for scabies in the armed forces and among the civilian population for the past sixty years or so, and attempts to show that some major or minor war is responsible for the rises in incidence which have apparently occurred from time to time. Where Friedman is unable to find a war on which to put the blame he is always able to discover some sort of punitive expedition or even a function like the Buffalo Exposition of 1902 and the St. Louis Exposition of 1904 with which to connect an otherwise inexplicable rise in the incidence of scabies !

Of two facts concerning the incidence of scabies there is no doubt—the disease was very common during the war of 1914–18 and it has become very common during the present war. Transmission within the armed forces is usually blamed for both of these epidemics. Actually, as has been shown in an earlier chapter, at the present day scabies is very rarely transmitted within the Services. Large numbers of sailors, soldiers, and airmen are found to be suffering from the disease, but this is merely because they are the only section of the population which is subject to regular medical examinations. Careful investigation soon reveals that far more cases of scabies in the Services are contracted from civilian contacts than *vice versa*.

The present distressingly high incidence of scabies might well have arisen if there had been no war at all ; this contention is supported by the fact that the rise which coincided with the war of 1914–18 was equally severe in neutral and belligerent countries. In Britain in 1918 scabies was exceedingly common, but it decreased to a very low level indeed by 1925. For the next five years it remained uncommon, though a slight increase in cases was noticeable.[1] From 1930 to 1935 a considerable increase took place, but even by the latter date it is unlikely that in the whole of Britain more than 0·1 per cent. of the population was affected. After 1935 the disease started to increase much more rapidly, and by 1937 and 1938 it was causing considerable concern to the authorities throughout the country. By the date of the outbreak of the war in September 1939 it is probable that nearly 1 per cent. of the population was infected with scabies. Since that date the disease has got considerably worse and it seems probable that in large sections of the community a degree of infestation as high as 5 per cent. exists ; the average for the country as a whole is perhaps in the region of 2 per cent. This

---

[1] Data prior to 1930 have been given by A. M. H. Gray, and refer to London school-children only ; data after 1930 include these and also other records for children and adults in many areas in Britain.

war-time increase would appear to be mainly the continuation of a trend which was clearly visible long before the outbreak of hostilities. That there has been epidemic scabies during two major wars is probably mainly a coincidence. The epidemic might have taken place anyhow. It is not improbable, however, that war-time conditions have done something to aggravate the situation.

Historical records indicate that scabies has been known throughout the history of mankind. The disease was common in Palestine in Biblical times and Hebra and others have suggested that a good deal of the so-called ' leprosy ' was only an infection with *Sarcoptes*. In the Middle Ages scabies was included among the eight common diseases. It is not surprising that scabies was so common, but what is difficult to explain is why it was not even more widespread, for social conditions were ideal for transmission. All the evidence at our disposal suggests that at all times the incidence went in waves ; it is easy to understand why the increase took place, but more difficult to understand why the incidence ever regressed, considering the inefficiency of the treatment usually given.

Most diseases which exhibit periodic fluctuations in their incidence do so largely because they confer some sort of immunity, either temporary or permanent, on those that recover from them. A disease introduced into a community that has not suffered from it previously spreads rapidly, and only decreases in incidence when a sufficient proportion of susceptible individuals have been rendered immune usually by recovery from an attack. The disease may then disappear from this population, or it may continue as a comparatively rare complaint. Another epidemic will not arise until a large non-immune population has arisen, either by loss of the temporary immunity received from the last attack, or else (if the immunity is more lasting) when a substantial fraction of the population has been replaced by new individuals. An attack of scabies does not confer anything like an absolute immunity. Many individuals have suffered from numerous attacks, and others have been infected for many years at a stretch (hence popular names for the disease like 'the seven years' itch'). Nevertheless in a considerable proportion of cases something like an immunity to a permanent infestation with *Sarcoptes* arises, for the individual becomes so greatly sensitised to the mite that his reaction shortly after infection is sufficient to cause it to be scratched out of its burrow and destroyed (see p. 26). Furthermore, scabies will only spread rapidly through a community which contains numerous unconscious carriers. The carrier in scabies is the person who has never had the disease before and who, though he may have many parasites, has not yet developed any sensitivity or itching sensations. For a period in their infection, every person who develops scabies can act as an unconscious carrier. Under present-day conditions, where efficient methods of treatment exist, once the disease has become common enough to render the population 'scabies conscious' vigorous action is likely to be taken by both patients and the authorities, and this also will tend to reduce the incidence.

The reasons given in the last paragraph hardly give a simple and clear-cut account of definite reasons why scabies sometimes increases and sometimes decreases in its incidence. The cumulative results of the several causes suggested may well be sufficient to account for what happens. On the other hand it is not unlikely that there are many other facts about *Sarcoptes* which are as yet imperfectly understood, and which have important effects on the incidence of the disease. Because scabies is caused by an arthropod which is large enough to be visible to the naked eye, one tends to think that everything about the disease and its incidence should be much more easily understood than in the case of diseases caused by microscopic and ultra microscopic organisms. Probably the causes of fluctuation in scabies are as complex as those of other diseases ; we are far from a full knowledge of the causes of the cycles of epidemics in any human disease.

There is some evidence to show that there is a seasonal incidence in scabies, and that the disease is at its lowest level in summer, rising in autumn and winter, to fall off again the following spring. This might be explained by the habit of people sleeping more in contact with one another for warmth during the cold parts of the year. Also most people wash less in winter than in summer and although this may have little effect on the *Sarcoptes* it may encourage secondary infection, and it frequently is this which causes the disease to be diagnosed. It should be remembered, however, that the symptoms of scabies generally take many weeks to develop, so that it is difficult to relate the cases treated at any centre on one particular day with seasonal changes in climatic conditions.

Scabies attacks all ages and both sexes, but at different periods different sections of the population have suffered most. In the 1860's in Vienna, Hebra found the disease was seven times as common in young males as in females, and he attributed this to the custom by which several apprentices slept together in the same bed. At present the disease is very common among children in Britain, and among young adults females appear to be twice as commonly affected as males. The high incidence in young females may partly be because they are most concerned with looking after children ; young women also share beds to a greater extent than do men. The high incidence in females compared with males is not necessarily explained by greater sexual promiscuity under present-day conditions. The high incidence in children is partly explained by scabies being a disease which spreads through families, particularly when they are overcrowded. Unfortunately most large families are compelled by economic motives to live under badly overcrowded conditions, ideal for the transmission of *Sarcoptes*.

CHAPTER VII

THE PREVENTION OF SCABIES

THE prevention of scabies is both a personal and a social problem. First, one wishes to know what individuals should be advised to do to avoid contracting the disease. Secondly, what steps should be taken by public health authorities to keep scabies under control.

In the past it has commonly been believed that a person who keeps himself reasonably clean is unlikely to contract scabies. Recent experience of those who have to deal with many cases of the disease does not support this idea, for many cases of infection have been seen in individuals of irreproachable personal hygiene. Experiments have been made with volunteers who have been infected with *Sarcoptes* and then subjected to daily baths ; the parasites attacking their bodies have increased in numbers as rapidly as in the case of other individuals who have had no baths for periods of up to two months. The mite, burrowing in the skin, does not seem to be at all adversely affected by ordinary washing. Vigorous use of a scrubbing brush will sometimes dislodge the parasite, but this does not occur as a rule until blood has been drawn. This explains why the finger nails are so much more efficient at removing the parasites than a scrubbing brush. It is not at all uncommon to see a person who has scratched himself until he has started bleeding, and the attention of the nails tends to be concentrated on the burrow containing the *Sarcoptes*. A nailbrush is seldom used with such vigour or accuracy.

When a mite first starts to burrow it takes about

an hour to dig into the cuticle. During that period it may well be removed by vigorous washing, but if this digging-in process occurs in bed the burrows will be well established before such an attack is likely. The immature stages are to be found comparatively superficially, and some will probably be removed by bathing, but the normal mortality during development is so great that there is no appreciable effect on the mite population. Mites certainly burrow readily into really clean skin ; it is possible that if the cuticle is filthy it may offer a less favourable harbourage to the parasite.

If cleanliness is of no avail, what steps should be taken to avoid infection with *Sarcoptes* ? Scabies is most likely to be avoided if one does not come into prolonged and intimate contact with some person suffering from the disease. Ordinary social contacts and even living in the same house with scabietic persons will probably not frequently transmit the disease. We have seen that it is possible to become infected by using a bed recently vacated by a scabies patient, but that this is unusual. There is little risk from an hotel bed ; even where the common, but unpleasant, custom of simply ironing and not washing bed-linen after one guest has used it is practised, it is unlikely that any acari will survive this treatment. It is unwise to put on unwashed underclothing used previously by an infected person, but this is hardly a common custom practised among cleanly persons of any social class. Communal blankets used by firewatchers offer some risk, but again it is probably a small one only, in the region of one chance in several thousands. Any adult should be practically certain of avoiding scabies. unless his children are unfortunate enough to contract the disease, if he exercises reasonable care in regard to those with whom he comes in intimate contact. It must be remembered that it is possible to become infected by sleeping together with someone who has not yet developed any clinical symptoms of scabies.

Scabies prevention, from the point of view of public health authorities, must be treated in two ways. A short-term policy must be pursued to deal with the present conditions and to try to control the number of cases which may arise ; a long-term policy should be aimed at producing conditions under which a further epidemic is unlikely.

The essence of the short-term policy, to deal with present conditions, is to have the public educated so that as soon as they have reason to suspect that a member of their household is infected, proper medical advice is sought, and further, that the advice is taken. But it will do more harm than good if the doctors and medical officers concerned are not able to make their diagnosis with certainty and if proper facilities for treatment are not available.

The question of the method of treatment is dealt with in detail in the next chapter. It has often been assumed that it is as important to deal with all fomites as with the persons of infected individuals. Experimental work detailed in an earlier chapter shows that this is not true and that although scabies can be transmitted by fomites this transmission is unlikely. Further, the layer of medicament which covers the body after anti-scabies treatment serves efficiently to disinfest any garments with which it comes in contact. If facilities for disinfestation are readily available it might be foolish not to use them, but there is no doubt that highly satisfactory results can be obtained with proper treatment and no dis-infestation whatsoever.

If fomites are of comparatively minor importance, too much importance can hardly be paid to the treatment of 'contacts.' Scabies is a disease of families, and particularly where there are small children it usually affects in some degree every member of a household. Whenever possible a whole household should be treated at the same time, particularly if the members are living under overcrowded conditions, irrespective of whether or not every member has developed clinical symptoms. In the past, where the treatment of the school children has often been the responsibility of the school medical authority (probably under the control of the county council) and the treatment of the younger children, adolescents, and adults has been the responsibility of the local health department, and where it has been impossible to bring pressure on reluctant patients, the whole state of affairs has been most unsatisfactory. The majority of those concerned with scabies believe that really satisfactory steps against the disease will only be possible if legislation goes forward to make it a notifiable disease,[1] but in the meantime the Scabies Order, 1941, which gives a medical officer of health powers to examine and treat any person suspected of being a ' scabies contact ', is a step in the right direction.

Social conditions are of considerable importance in the question of scabies. Overcrowding is one of the most potent causes of spread, and so any steps to improve housing would also help to combat future scabies epidemics. Only a very small proportion of the inhabitants, children or adults, in this country sleep in beds by themselves ; a universal introduction of the single bed would do more than anything else to put a stop to the spread of scabies ! (This can hardly be put forward as a practical policy.)

Rigorous segregation of cases of scabies, including

---

[1] Scabies may now be made notifiable in any area in which the local authority is considered to have the necessary facilities for diagnosis and treatment.

exclusion from schools and factories, is a step of doubtful usefulness unless these measures ensure that efficient treatment is given immediately. With modern methods of treatment it should be possible for any cases detected at school or in the factory to be treated the same day and they need not miss a further hour of school or work. It is unlikely that even before treatment they are any great danger to their schoolfellows and colleagues, and certainly after a single treatment with an efficient medicament any danger that did exist will be removed. A frequent cause for delay in treatment is the difficulty in making administrative arrangements for collecting and disinfesting fomites ; in my opinion, if difficulties caused by this are such as to delay treatment by as much as one day, it would be far wiser to forego the disinfestation.

5

CHAPTER VIII

THE TREATMENT OF SCABIES

THERE are rapid and efficient remedies which will cure every case of scabies without the slightest difficulty. When one realizes how very easy it is to kill all the mites invading the human cuticle, one is amazed at the difficulties which arise in the treatment of this disease. The whole secret of successful cure depends on efficient diagnosis. The average error in the diagnosis of scabies is in the region of 25 per cent., and as long as this continues it depends mainly on chance whether the relapse rate in a treatment centre is as high as 25 per cent. or as low as nil. It is significant that Hebra, who, a hundred years ago, treated many thousand cases of scabies with sulphur ointment, found a practically negligible relapse rate ; he was thoroughly familiar with *Sarcoptes* and so is unlikely to have had any difficulties in making a correct diagnosis. In more recent years the Danish worker Kissmeyer was another who was thoroughly familiar with the features of human scabies ; using benzyl benzoate to treat 8000 cases he obtained a cure in almost every instance. Recent work has shown that as compared with other popular methods of treatment these two, sulphur ointment and benzyl benzoate, can be relied upon to give excellent results when properly applied, whereas most other so-called remedies are of much less value.

Unfortunately, in many cases of scabies, it is necessary not only to kill the invading *Sarcoptes*, but also to cure the skin of more serious secondary infection. There has been much confusion between the direct effects of the acari and of secondary bacterial infection and the usual belief has been that where the body is covered with pustular lesions this is a ' severe ' case of scabies and therefore more difficult to cure than a case free from pyodermia. The secondarily infected case will certainly take longer to heal completely, but it is not by any means necesarily more difficult to exterminate the *Sarcoptes* (of which incidentally there may be very few living individuals present). And most of the medicaments used to kill the acari are not of much value in curing pyodermia, in fact as they are skin irritants they may have an adverse effect. Secondary infection must be treated as such and treated by measures suitable to the nature of the condition in each individual.

There is no such thing as a resistant case of scabies. If the treatment is really competently applied, every case should be readily cured. So called ' resistant cases ' may be individuals who are constantly being reinfected. More likely they are not actually infected with *Sarcoptes* at all, at any rate after the first treatment. Either they are cases in which the itching persists, as it not uncommonly does, for a considerable period after the scabies is cured, or else persistent secondary infection is being described as persistent active scabies.

(A) THE TREATMENT OF THE PARASITIC INFECTION

The object of any medicament is to kill all stages of *Sarcoptes* as rapidly as possible, with the minimum of discomfort and inconvenience to the patient. In addition, to be widely used the medicament must be reasonably inexpensive.

It has generally been found that the thoroughness and efficiency with which a method has been applied

is as important as the choice of the method itself.
Many workers have thought that preparatory treatment, including bathing and scrubbing, is of para-
mount importance. Treatment orderlies have been
encouraged to scrub their patients with extreme
vigour, often to the great discomfort of the patient
and to the detriment of his epidermis. It is
usual, at present, to recommend a thorough bath
and the patient is advised to rub the affected areas
with a flannel but not to use a scrubbing brush.
Experimental work has shown that equally efficient
cures are obtained when the bath is omitted, though,
as so many scabies patients are rather dirty, it is
advisable to give the bath for hygienic reasons. But
care and thoroughness in applying the medicament is
necessary for successful treatment.

A brief description is given below of the majority
of methods which have been popular in the treatment
of scabies. The Table summarises the power of
the different medicaments to kill *Sarcoptes*. The
methods   have   been   assessed   by   examining
patients 24 hours after one application of the
medicament, when the acari have been removed
and examined to discover the proportion which has
been killed. Experiments indicate that a medicament
which kills the adult acari will be effective against all
stages :

    (1) *Sulphur Ointment.* B.P. sulphur ointment con-
           taining 10 per cent. sulphur is rubbed over
           the whole surface of the body. Approxi-
           mately 3 oz. is required for each application.
           The method is a very messy one, but self-
           treatment is possible and excellent results
           may be obtained. A much more pleasant
           ointment may be produced by incorporating
           the sulphur in a vanishing cream base ; it
           appears to be equally effective.

(2) *Marcussen's Ointment.* This ointment contains a mixture of unstable polysulphides and is said to have the advantage that one application will cure human scabies within 24 hours. Experimental work supports this claim, but it must be remembered that ordinary sulphur ointment is nearly as effective.

(3) *Flowers of Sulphur.* Scabies is frequently treated simply by dusting flowers of sulphur over the body of the patient and inside his underclothing and sleeping garments. This method is very inefficient, killing only a small proportion of the parasites and being very liable to cause a sulphur dermatitis before giving a satisfactory cure.

(4) *Sodium Thiosulphate and Hydrochloric Acid.* In this method the patient is first painted with a strong solution of hypo, which is then followed by some acid (*i.e.* hydrochloric) which releases the sulphur together with a certain amount of sulphur dioxide. The method is little more effective than dusting with flowers of sulphur and there seems little reason for continuing its use.

(5) *Sulphur Soaps.* Various sulphur lather preparations have been tried in the treatment of scabies. A thin film of sulphur particles is deposited all over the body of the patient. It appears to have comparatively little effect against the parasites.

(6) *Sulphur taken Internally.* Some investigators have reported that cases of scabies that cannot be cured by other methods have responded rapidly to sulphur taken internally. Experimental work has shown that even if the largest dose which can be con-

sumed without causing severe physical discomfort (*i.e.* approximately 10 g. daily) is taken, the parasites of an existing infection are quite unharmed and no protection is given against a fresh infection.

(7) *Derris Root Lotion.* Powdered derris root is widely used as an insecticide. A lotion made by mixing 4 oz. of derris root with 1 gallon of water containing a small quantity of soap flakes, has been advised in the treatment of scabies. It has much less effect than sulphur ointment and its use is not recommended.

(8) *Rotenone Emulsion.* The main active principal of derris root is rotenone and various preparations containing this substance have been used against scabies. After one application 25 per cent. of the mites remain alive, and a number of applications is required to give results comparable with those of sulphur ointment. Furthermore, rotenone emulsions are very liable to give rise to serious dermatitis and so their use is not recommended.

(9) *Pyrethrum.* A number of pyrethrum extracts which are very effective against insects were found to be considerably less satisfactory in the treatment of human scabies. The use of pyrethrum compounds against this disease is not therefore to be recommended.

(10) *Betanaphthol.* Various ointments containing betanaphthol have been used, but they again appear to be considerably less efficient than sulphur ointment.

(11) *Lethane.* Organic thiocyanates such as lethane are very effective against lice, but a 2 per cent. solution in medicinal paraffin, which is

as strong as can be supported by the skin of most individuals without causing considerable discomfort, only kills about two thirds of the parasites.

(12) *Dimethyl-diphenylene Disulphide* (*Dimethyl-thianthrene*). This substance, formerly marketed as *Mitigal*, which is a golden-yellowish, oily liquid, is painted undiluted over the surface of the body. It does not appear to cause dermatitis and is very effective against *Sarcoptes*. It is, unfortunately, very expensive and therefore unsuited to treating large numbers of patients. The liquid can be diluted with medicinal paraffin and even in as weak a solution as one containing 10 per cent., it is still effective against human scabies. Under war conditions both the dimethyl-diphenylene disulphide and paraffin are scarce, which probably rules out this method for present use.

(13) *Benzyl Benzoate* has been used in many forms for the treatment of scabies and emulsions in water are probably the most satisfactory. They do not often cause dermatitis, they are comparatively painless, even in the case of badly abraided skin, and they do not soil underclothing or bedding. Formulae for making up benzyl benzoate emulsions are given in the Appendix. Incidentally, where stearic acid and triethanolamine are used to make the emulsion, it is practically painless even with babies ; lanette wax occasionally causes more severe discomfort.

A comparison of the efficiency of different methods used in the treatment of scabies to kill *Sarcoptes* after one application of the medicament.

Treatment.				*Mites Killed.*
				per cent.
Sulphur ointment B.P.	.	.	.	97–100
Marcussen's ointment	.	.	.	100
Flowers of sulphur	.	.	.	15
Thiosulphate—HCl	.	.	.	25
Sulphur soap	.	.	.	17
Internal sulphur	.	.	.	0
Derris root lotion	.	.	.	73
Rotenone emulsion	.	.	.	76
Pyrethrum preparation	.	.	.	59–94
Betanaphthol	.	.	.	82
Lethane	.	.	.	68
Dimethyl-diphenylene Disulphide	.	.	100
Benzyl Benzoate (20 per cent. emulsion in water)	99.9

The Notes and Table given above show that four substances, sulphur ointment, Marcussen's ointment, dimethyl-diphenylene disulphide, and benzyl benzoate are efficient medicaments in the treatment of human scabies. Under present-day conditions it would be advisable to rely on two of these only, sulphur ointment and benzyl benzoate, as they contain the substances most easily obtainable. In most cases benzyl benzoate is probably the preferable medicament, and it has the advantage of not containing large quantities of fatty substances, as are used in the bases for sulphur ointment. It also does not soil clothing and bedding, an important consideration in these days of rationing. If skilled orderlies are available there is no doubt that the benzyl benzoate should be used, but sulphur ointment still offers some advantages for self-treatment. The following notes suggest the methods which have been found efficient in treating the disease :

(a) Treatment with Benzyl Benzoate

If bathing facilities are available the patient should be given a bath, but lack of bathing facilities should not prevent treatment being carried out as this is not greatly affected by preliminary washing. If the patient is bathed he is thoroughly dried and then the benzyl benzoate emulsion is applied, using an ordinary flat paint brush, about 2 inches in diameter, all over the body from the neck downwards. It is important that the whole body should be painted and to obtain success conscientious orderlies, properly supervized, are required. At the end of the painting the body is allowed to dry (this takes 5 to 10 minutes in a warm room) after which the patient dresses. To allow for inefficiency in treatment and other possible sources of failure, it is advisable to prescribe two paintings, either on successive days or within one week, but where the treatment is performed really conscientiously, over 95 per cent. of cures are to be expected with one treatment only. Where facilities exist for sterilising clothes and bedding, these may be treated, but it is unlikely that omission to do this will have any appreciable effect on the ultimate result. An efficient treatment orderly is worth a hundred sterilisers !

(b) Treatment with Sulphur Ointment

With sulphur ointment it is probably advisable to give two inunctions, either on succeeding days or within a period of a week. Approximately 3 ozs. of the ointment is rubbed into the skin, covering the whole surface of the body. It is usually deemed advisable to have a bath before the first application, but no bath should be taken between the two inunctions. Two inunctions should give a cure even if no bath is available.

(B) THE TREATMENT OF SECONDARY INFECTION

One, or at most two, applications of benzyl benzoate lotion or sulphur ointment can be relied upon to exterminate the *Sarcoptes*, but unfortunately, in many cases, secondary pathological skin conditions remain, which require further treatment. Incidentally, even when little secondary infection exists, the skin cannot be expected to be completely normal immediately after a treatment which is complete within 24 hours. It has been usual to continue treatment for several days, but actually the skin should heal as well, or better, with no further scabies treatment.

The writer is not a dermatologist and is therefore not competent to advise on the treatment of secondary infection. The following notes are included for the sake of completeness :

The first essential is that the skin of the patient should be really clean. When secondary infection is common, bathing facilities are almost essential at any scabies treatment centre, even although *Sarcoptes* itself can be satisfactorily dealt with by means of benzyl benzoate without preliminary bathing. The patient should soak for 5 or 10 minutes ; soap should be used, but soft soap (particularly the war-time substitute which itself is apt to cause dermatitis) is better avoided. The skin may be rubbed with a cloth or flannel, *not* with a scrubbing brush.

An ordinary bath, as described above, followed by a satisfactory anti-scabies treatment with no special measures against the sepsis, not infrequently has surprisingly good results against both conditions, but it is generally advisable to take further steps against the secondary condition.

If there are many crusts, these should be removed first of all. Various treatments are commonly used, for instance, boracic fomentations or starch poultices, formulae for which will be found in all text books of dermatology.

After removal of crusts, the underlying sepsis may be treated in various ways, and different specialists are by no means in agreement as to the best methods. Dilute mercury ointment, 1 in 1000 acriflavine lotion and gentian violet all give good results on many patients, lotions being preferable to ointments when the impetigo is very moist. Preparations containing some of the sulphonamine compounds have given good results in the hands of some workers and appear to give the most rapid results in very serious cases. Widespread follicular pustules often respond to the application of calamine lotion ; in the more resistant cases a 2 per cent. solution of silver nitrate may be used. In a centre where very large numbers must be treated, and where the medical officer cannot give much individual attention to every case, it is advisable to select one of the above treatments to be given in the first instance to all patients whose condition is not sufficiently serious to require detention in hospital. Re-examination after a week will reveal which patients do and do not respond satisfactorily and the latter can then have special treatment. Actually the majority of cases of serious secondary infection clear up remarkably easily, but a small minority prove very resistant to treatment. In these latter it is always advisable wherever possible to obtain the advice of a competent dermatologist.

Secondary eczema may be very troublesome. Often it clears with simple sedatives such as calamine lotion or calamine and zinc cream when the scabies has been cured, but at other times it continues in spite of every type of treatment, and this again is a problem which should have the individual attention of a dermatologist.

Finally it must be stated that excellent results are

not infrequently obtained under the most unlikely conditions. Children with severe sepsis are in some centres severely scrubbed by untrained personnel, and then liberally plastered with 10 per cent. sulphur ointment. In many the secondary infection clears up amazingly rapidly. I do not advocate, however, that these methods should be introduced where a more satisfactory form of treatment is possible. It may again be remarked that if it is possible to ensure 100 per cent. diagnosis of scabies in its early stages there will be no trouble with secondary infection.

CHAPTER IX

CONDITIONS WHICH MAY BE CONFUSED WITH SCABIES

SEVERAL other diseases are frequently confused with scabies ; about 25 per cent. of patients sent in to one treatment centre were found to be suffering from other complaints which included pediculosis corporis, pediculosis pubis, eczema of various types, dermatitis due to a variety of causes, papular urticaria, generalized coccogenic folliculitis, seborrhoea, and even syphilis. Certain of these diseases (*e.g.* syphilis and pediculosis pubis) are not uncommonly found in conjunction with scabies. As has been stated many times in earlier sections of this book, the one really satisfactory way of diagnosing scabies is to discover the parasite ; to exclude scabies one must be certain there are no *Sarcoptes* present. The following notes may give some additional assistance in preventing scabies being wrongly diagnosed :

Pediculosis corporis or infestation of the body by the louse *Pediculus humanus corporis*. The patient will probably complain of itching which is worst at night. A satisfactory diagnosis is only made if one or more lice can be discovered ; these insects are most likely to be found on the garments worn next to the skin, and not on the body itself. A good deal of difficulty in finding lice may be experienced, for many chronically lousy individuals only have half a dozen or so of the parasites on their persons. The typical linear scratch marks, frequently on the shoulder blades, chest, and other areas free from lesions in scabies, lead one to suspect lice. The nits or eggs are laid usually on the inner garments, particularly in the seams, and their presence may help diagnosis. Incidentally a lousy individual not infrequently has scabies as well.

Pediculosis capitis, or infestation of the head by the louse *Pediculus humanus capitis* is less likely to be confused with scabies, but a high proportion of female scabies patients have lousy heads. The lice are seldom found away from the head, but in very heavy infestations a few may be found among the clothes. Incidentally it is unwise to pass any female's head as free from lice unless it has been combed with a fine comb for at least 5 minutes without finding any insect.

Pediculosis pubis, or infestation with *Phthirus pubis*, the crab louse. This insect is usually confined to the hairs of the pubis and the axillae, though in hairy individuals it may be found on the general surface of the body. The itching caused by the crab louse is usually confined to the infested areas, and the discovery of the insects, which often evade discovery by the way they cling firmly and almost immovably to the skin, confirms the diagnosis. Typical ' blue spots,' usually about 3 mm. in diameter in the skin of the affected areas, appear to be caused by the bite of *Phthirus*; their presence is often noticed before the lice are observed. The greyish nits stuck to the hairs are also a useful diagnostic sign. I have several times seen crab lice, body lice and scabies simultaneously on the same patient.

Fleas and Bugs in billets may sometimes give symptoms which are confused with *Sarcoptes* infestation, particularly in the ' scabies-conscious.' It is seldom possible to find these insects, particularly the bed-bug *Cimex*, on the persons of their victims, and it may be necessary to make a careful examination of the house property concerned.

Urticaria papulosa in children may often be confused with scabies, particularly when scratching has led to much secondary infection. If no burrows can be found, if the eruption is mostly confined to the lower limbs, buttocks and forearms, and if there is evidence that the condition is not contagious (*i.e.* another child who sleeps in the same bed as the patient is not affected) then it is probable that the trouble is papular urticaria rather than scabies. Papular urticaria also tends to be a disease which recurs at fairly long intervals during which the patient is free from all symptoms.

Eczema is sometimes treated as scabies ; on the other hand eczematous symptoms will frequently mask a primary infection of scabies. If an eczematous rash has the distribution usually associated with scabies, it is always as well to make redoubled efforts to ensure that *Sarcoptes* is not the underlying cause.

Occupational dermatitis may be mistaken for scabies ; more frequently scabies is mistaken for an occupational dermatitis and compensation is claimed by the patient.

Treatment dermatitis due in particular to self medication, particularly with sulphur ointment, causes much trouble in scabies treatment centres. One characteristic of this condition is persistent itching very like active scabies. It is not unusual, as a result of unskilled treatment, to have a dermatitis caused by over-treatment of one part of the body with living *Sarcoptes* which have been neglected. Unless the person making the examination is familiar with the parasite he will be unlikely to recognize this.

Coccogenic folliculitis. This condition may arise

secondarily to scabies, and may then clear when the primary infection is cured. On the other hand a widespread folliculitis occurs not infrequently without any suspicion of scabies. Unfortunately in either case the general distribution of the rash may be the same, and once more a satisfactory diagnosis depends on the discovery or otherwise of *Sarcoptes*.

Syphilis. A primary sore on the penis is sometimes confused with a burrow of *Sarcoptes* ; the chancre may even develop in the site of a scratched-out burrow, for scabies and syphilis not infrequently occur simultaneously. It is most unusual in scabies to find a single well-defined penile lesion with no other signs on other parts of the body. The secondary syphilitic rash should seldom be confused with scabies, particularly as the lesions do not itch and generally affect those areas of the body unaffected by scabies.

Persistent itching with consequent scratch lesions is often found for some time after a successful treatment. In cases like this, repeated treatment with subsequent dermatitis is common unless the effects of the medicaments on the parasites are carefully noted.

CHAPTER X

OTHER MITES OF MEDICAL AND VETERINARY IMPORTANCE

In addition to *Sarcoptes scabiei* var. *hominis* there are various other mites of medical importance. There is also a number of species of importance in veterinary practice ; some of these mites occasionally find their way on to man, and they are among the miscellaneous specimens sent to the laboratory as the ' cause ' of a variety of skin troubles.

The term ' mite ' is given to a miscellaneous collection of animals. They are all Arachnida and belong to the order Acarina. This order, the Acarina, comprises those creatures known as ticks and mites. The ticks form a more or less uniform group—the suborder Mesostigmata—and includes a number of species of medical importance such as *Ornithodoros* and *Dermacentor*. The mites, on the other hand, are members of at least four sub-orders which bear little resemblance to one another. A simplified classification which indicates the zoological position of some of the mites of medical and veterinary importance is given below. Fig. 10 gives some idea of their general appearance. The animals shown in the figure are all drawn to scale, and their size, as compared with *Sarcoptes*, may be estimated in relation to the scale shown, and to the fact that the adult *Notoedrus* (Fig. 10c) is approximately the same size as the larva of *Sarcoptes* (see Fig. 2b).

PHYLUM ARTHROPODA

CLASS HEXAPODA (Insects).
CLASS CRUSTACEA (Crabs, cyclops, etc.).
6

CLASS ARACHNIDA.
        ORDER ARANEAE (Spiders).
        ORDER SCORPIONES (Scorpions).
        ORDER ACARINA (Ticks and mites).
                Sarcoptes.
                Trombicula.
                Demodex.
                Aleurobius.
                Pediculoides.
                Notoedrus.
                Otodectes.
                Psoroptes.

Sarcoptes.

Some mention has been made in an earlier chapter of the different varieties of *Sarcoptes scabiei* which occur on most species of domestic animals. No constant morphological distinctions for the *Sarcoptes* from the different mammals have been described, but there seem to be physiological differences, and each mammal has its own 'biological race.' Man can be infected by the *Sarcoptes* from domestic animals, but the infestation does not appear to be permanent and dies out in a few weeks. The view that Norwegian or Crusted Scabies is due to an infestation of man by parasites from animals is probably incorrect. The main difference between human and animal scabies is that when *Sarcoptes* occurs on domestic animals, instead of a dozen or so adult females, many thousands are commonly found to occur. It is because the parasites are so numerous that veterinary students and others coming in close contact with animals can pick up sufficient mites to give appreciable symptoms in a transient infestation.

In man it is the active finger nails of the host which keep down the parasite population, and the reason why mites are so numerous in animal scabies may well be that they do not possess appendages so well suited to the removal of these enemies. It is also possible that when numbers of mites similar to those present in most cases of human scabies occur on a hairy mammal they frequently pass undetected.

Trombicula

It is characteristic of the Acarina that the stage which emerges from the egg is a six-legged larva. In many species the larva lives quite a different sort of life from the later stages; for instance, many larvae attack mammals and suck blood, whereas the later stages in the life-history of the same species are entirely vegetarian. It has proved impossible to breed the majority of those blood-sucking larvae to maturity, and there is a good deal of doubt as to which larvae correspond to the adults which are commonly collected in nature. As a result the systematics of the group are somewhat obscure and the names attributed to the larvae must be considered as provisional.

Trombicula autumnalis is the common ' harvest bug ' (Fig. 10a) found in various parts of Britain. It is particularly common in autumn, when it attacks the legs of those working in fields and gardens. As will be seen from the figure, the harvest bug, even in its larval stage is fully as large as an adult of *Sarcoptes*, and the adults of these *Trombiculae* may be more than 5 mm. in length. When feeding on man the larva remains attached for a considerable period, and if it is forcibly removed the mouth-parts may be left behind in the flesh to serve as a centre for serious inflammation and sepsis. Less serious results are usual if the mite is allowed to gorge and drop off naturally, but even then the site of the bite may be intensely irritating. The common British species are not as a rule more than a nuisance, though they may cause serious discomfort to gardeners and agricultural workers. In other parts of the world, however, larvae of a similar nature are of considerable medical importance. In Japan, Formosa, and the Far East generally, Japanese river fever or pseudo-typhus is believed to be caused by a virus carried by a species of *Trombicula*.

Aleurobius, Pediculoides, etc.

These mites are found living among grain and other stored food products. They may become exceedingly numerous and cause serious loss of foodstuffs. Though they are unable to parasitize man their presence is often responsible for setting up a severe dermatitis in those handling infested materials. The disease known as ' grocer's itch ' may be caused by this type of mite, though various forms of dermatitis due to sensitization to substances frequently handled are also described as ' grocer's itch.' Fig. 10*b* shows a specimen of *Aleurobius*. Incidentally, the well-known cheese-mite is a species of *Aleurobius*.

Notoedrus.

This mite (Fig. 10*c*) is superficially similar in appearance to *Sarcoptes*, and has sometimes been described under the name of *Sarcoptes minor* ; it is about half the size of the human itch mite. *Notoedrus* attacks the cat, rabbit, and other domestic animals ; a transient infection may occur in persons who handle heavily infested animals.

Demodex.

The mite *Demodex folliculorum* (Fig. 10*d*) occurs in the sebaceous glands of man. It is very widespread, but is mainly a commensal and causes no trouble to its host. *Demodex* has, with little positive evidence, been accused of causing acne, leprosy, and cancer of

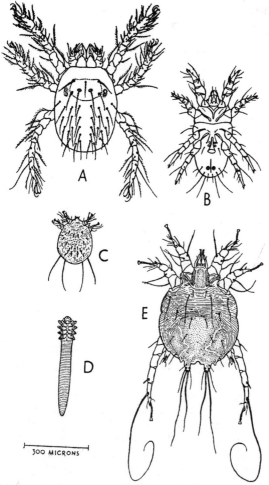

Fig. 10. Mites of medical and veterinary importance.
(a) *Trombicula autumnalis* (harvest bug). (b) *Aleurobius*.
(c) *Notoedrus*. (d) *Demodex*. (e) *Psoroptes*.

the skin. *Demodex* in animals causes a serious follicular mange, and it is possible that the species from
dogs and horses may occasionally cause eruptions on
the skin of man.

Otodectes.

Otodectes commonly attacks domestic cats; in
some cities the majority are infected. The mite
lives in the ears, and characteristic symptoms are a
constant shaking of the head and the presence of
black, scaly masses inside the pinna. Numerous
mites can usually be found among the scales. *Otodectes* is not recorded as attacking man.

Psoroptes.

Psoroptic mange or ‘ sheep scab ’ causes severe loss
to farmers in most parts of the world. *Psoroptes*
(Fig. 10e) also attacks other domestic animals and
causes a serious type of mange. Man has occasionally
been affected but the attack is only of a very transitory
nature.

APPENDIX

THE following miscellaneous formulae may be of some value to those interested in scabies :

(1) Berlese's Fluid

This preparation can be used for mounting mites or pieces of tissue containing burrows, etc. It serves as a fixing, clearing, and mounting medium, so that the use of different concentrations of alcohol, xylol, etc., are unnecessary. The formula is as follows :

Water	20 mils.
Chloral hydrate	160 g.
Gum arabic	15 g.
Glucose syrup (or domestic golden syrup)	10 mils.
Glacial acetic acid	5 g.

Dissolve the chloral hydrate slowly in the water (this is a tedious and troublesome process) add the acetic acid, which may help the last part of the chloral hydrate to dissolve. Next add the gum arabic, well powdered and finally add the syrup.

Acari and pieces of tissue may be mounted on slides in this medium and covered with a cover-slip. In a dry climate a permanent preparation is made without further treatment, though the slides will take some weeks to dry. Under moist conditions it may be advisable to ring the slides with gold size and finish off with black asphaltum.

(2) Benzyl Benzoate Emulsion

Emulsions of benzyl benzoate in water are very easy to make, and all forms appear equally effective,

provided they contain at least 20 per cent. of benzyl
benzoate. Reliable proprietary brands of benzyl
benzoate are on the market, mostly at a retail price
of approximately 4s. per 4 oz. When the constituents
are bought in bulk any of the emulsions described
below can be made up at less than 4d. for 4 oz. The
proprietary brands show no advantages over the
article as made up by a reliable dispenser. In case
any emulsifying agent is scarce, three different
formulae are given :

(a) Benzyl benzoate	.	.	200 mils.
Stearic acid	.	.	20 g.
Triethanolamine	.	.	6 mils.
Water to produce	.	.	1000 mils.

Heat together the benzyl benzoate and stearic
acid until the latter is dissolved. Mix the triethanolamine with the water and then pour this into the
warm benzyl benzoate-stearic acid mixture and stir.
This preparation has the advantage that it appears
impossible not to make a good emulsion and the liquid
is much the least painful of all the emulsions on a
tender and abraided skin.

(b) Benzyl benzoate	.	.	200 mils.
Lanette wax S.X.	.	.	10 g.
Water	.	.	.	800 mils.

Melt the lanette wax on a water-bath, add the
benzyl benzoate and heat the mixture to a temperature of between 60° and 70° C. Pour the mixture into
the water, previously heated to the same temperature
and stir until cold.

To make the emulsion according to the National
War Formulary the benzyl benzoate should be increased to 250 mils., the lanette wax to 20 g. and
the water decreased to 750 mils. We have found no

advantage in this higher concentration and the formula as given above is much more economical.

(c) Benzyl benzoate . . . . . 200 mils.
    1 per cent. solution of cellofas W.F.Z. . 800 mils.

Shake together to form an emulsion. Put through a cream-making machine or homogenizer.

INDEX

NoTE.—No direct references are given to either Scabies or *Sarcoptes*, as these would appear on every page. In this Index S. stands for *Sarcoptes*.